THE COMPLETE DIABETES REVERSAL COOKBOOK FOR BEGINNERS

A FLAVORFUL JOURNEY THROUGH DIABETES-FRIENDLY RECIPES FOR VIBRANT HEALTH

JEFF MARK

TABLE OF CONTENT

INTRODUCTION

There was Sarah, a vibrant soul who navigated life's daily adventures while silently wrestling with the challenges of diabetes. Her life revolved around insulin shots, blood sugar tests, and dietary restrictions. Despite her unwavering spirit, the constant battle with her health took a toll.

One serendipitous day, Sarah stumbled upon a diabetes cookbook while browsing through her local bookstore. Intrigued, she flipped through its pages, discovering a plethora of tantalizing recipes crafted specifically for individuals managing diabetes. The vibrant images and promising descriptions ignited a spark of hope within her.

Determined to change her approach to food and health, Sarah delved into the cookbook's contents with enthusiasm. She started experimenting with the recipes, gradually incorporating the book's guidance into her daily routine. She swapped processed snacks for homemade nutrient-packed alternatives, bid farewell to sugary indulgences, and welcomed colorful, wholesome meals into her life.

As weeks turned into months, something remarkable began to unfold. Sarah noticed gradual changes in her energy levels, mood, and, most significantly, her blood sugar readings. Her doctor, pleasantly surprised, witnessed the remarkable improvement and cautiously reduced her medication dosage.

Sarah's culinary journey became an adventure filled with new ingredients, innovative cooking techniques, and a newfound love for creating meals that were not just healthy but also delicious. She discovered the joy of preparing meals from scratch, relishing each bite with a newfound appreciation for the flavors of fresh produce, lean proteins, and smart carbohydrates.

Months passed, and Sarah's commitment to the cookbook's recipes became a way of life. With each passing day, her health blossomed. Her doctor, astounded by her progress, declared something Sarah had never imagined hearing: "Your diabetes is under control."

The transformative power of embracing a diabetes-friendly diet had not only improved Sarah's health but had also changed her perspective on food. She had found a sense of empowerment in making mindful choices, enjoying meals that not only nourished her body but also fed her soul.

Sarah's journey from reliance on medications to managing her health primarily through food was nothing short of a miracle. The diabetes cookbook, once just a collection of recipes, had become her guide to a life filled with vitality, flavor, and newfound freedom from the clutches of diabetes.

Her story spread hope among others facing similar health challenges. Sarah became an advocate, sharing her experience and the life-changing impact of embracing a diabetes-conscious diet. She proved that with dedication, knowledge, and a touch of culinary creativity, a cookbook could be a gateway to a healthier, brighter future.

And thus, Sarah's tale stood as a testament to the transformative potential of a well-crafted diabetes cookbook, inspiring countless others to embark on their own journeys towards better health and wellness.

Diabetes is a chronic metabolic disorder that affects how your body processes glucose, the primary source of energy for your cells. Whether you have been recently diagnosed or have been living with diabetes for some time, understanding the fundamentals of this condition is the first step towards effective management.

Living with diabetes is a journey that involves mindful choices, especially when it comes to food. Whether you're newly diagnosed or have been managing diabetes for years, understanding the impact of diet on blood sugar levels is crucial. This cookbook aims to be your companion, providing not just recipes but also knowledge and guidance to empower you in your daily culinary choices.

Food plays a pivotal role in managing diabetes. Every meal presents an opportunity to make choices that positively impact your health. This cookbook emphasizes a balanced approach, focusing on nutrient-dense, low-glycemic, and wholesome ingredients. By harnessing the power of fresh produce, lean proteins, and smart carbohydrates, these recipes aim to help stabilize blood sugar levels while tantalizing your taste buds.

GUIDELINES FOR COOKING WITH DIABETES

1. **Embrace Balanced Nutrition:**

- **Carbohydrate Management:** Monitor and manage carbohydrate intake as it directly affects blood sugar levels. Opt for complex carbohydrates with a low glycemic index, such as whole grains, legumes, and non-starchy vegetables.

- **Lean Proteins:** Incorporate lean proteins like skinless poultry, fish, tofu, legumes, and nuts into meals to promote satiety without affecting blood sugar significantly.

- **Healthy Fats:** Choose sources of healthy fats, such as avocados, olive oil, nuts, and seeds, while moderating the portion sizes to maintain a healthy weight.

2. **Mindful Meal Planning:**

- **Portion Control:** Pay attention to portion sizes to avoid overeating, which can impact blood sugar levels. To help you manage servings, use plates that are smaller.

- **Meal Timing:** Consistency in meal timing is key. Aim for regular mealtimes spaced evenly throughout the day to maintain stable blood sugar levels.

3. **Smart Ingredient Choices:**

- **Favor Fiber-Rich Foods:** Integrate high-fiber foods like fruits, vegetables, whole grains, and legumes into meals to help control blood sugar levels and promote digestive health.

- **Reduce Added Sugars:** Minimize the use of refined sugars and sweeteners in recipes. Instead, use natural sweeteners like stevia or opt for fruit as a sweetening agent.

- **Control Sodium Intake:** Monitor sodium levels to support heart health. Use herbs, spices, and other flavorings to season meals instead of salt.

4. **Cooking Techniques and Meal Preparation:**

- **Healthy Cooking Methods:** Choose healthier cooking methods like baking, grilling, steaming, or sautéing with minimal oil to reduce unnecessary fats in meals.

- **Preparation of Complete Meals:** Aim to create balanced meals that include a combination of protein, healthy fats, and fiber-rich carbohydrates to aid in better blood sugar regulation.

5. **Regular Monitoring and Adaptation:**

- **Monitor Blood Sugar Levels:** Keep track of blood sugar levels regularly, especially after meals, to understand how different foods affect your body and adjust your diet accordingly.

- **Work with a Healthcare Professional:** Consult with a registered dietitian or healthcare provider to tailor a meal plan specific to your needs and lifestyle.

6. **Stay Hydrated and Be Mindful:**

- **Stay Hydrated:** Drink plenty of water throughout the day to stay hydrated, support bodily functions, and aid in digestion.

- Eat mindfully by taking note of your hunger signals, chew your food carefully, and enjoy every taste. Better digestion and a reduction in overeating may result from doing this.

IMPORTANT OF DIET IN MANAGING DIABETES

Diet plays a pivotal role in the effective management of diabetes, providing individuals with a powerful tool to control blood sugar levels, enhance overall well-being, and reduce the risk of complications. A well-balanced and carefully planned diet can make a significant impact on managing diabetes and improving the quality of life for those living with this condition.

1. **Blood Sugar Regulation:** Proper nutrition helps regulate blood sugar levels, preventing spikes and crashes that can be detrimental for individuals with diabetes. Strategic carbohydrate choices and portion control contribute to maintaining stable glucose levels throughout the day.

2. **Weight Management:** Maintaining a healthy weight is crucial for individuals with diabetes, as excess weight can contribute to insulin resistance. A balanced diet, combined with regular physical activity, supports weight management and improves insulin sensitivity.

3. **Heart Health:** Heart disease is more common in those who have diabetes. A heart-healthy diet, rich in whole grains, fruits, vegetables, and lean proteins, helps manage cholesterol and blood pressure levels. Omega-3 fatty acids from sources like fatty fish and flaxseeds contribute to cardiovascular health.

4. **Prevention of Complications**: Consistent adherence to a diabetes-friendly diet can help prevent complications such as nerve damage, kidney disease, and eye problems. Antioxidant-rich foods, including fruits and vegetables, may provide protective benefits against oxidative stress associated with diabetes-related complications.

5. **Energy and Vitality:** Proper nutrition ensures a steady and sustained energy supply, combating fatigue and promoting overall vitality. Balanced meals with a mix of macronutrients provide essential nutrients for optimal bodily functions.

6. **Improved Insulin Sensitivity:** Certain foods, particularly those with a low glycemic index, can improve insulin sensitivity and assist the body in using insulin more effectively.

Including fiber-rich foods and whole grains in the diet supports stable blood sugar levels.

7. **Individualized Nutrition Plans:** Tailoring the diet to individual needs and preferences allows for a more sustainable and personalized approach to diabetes management. Consultation with healthcare professionals and registered dietitians can help create a customized nutrition plan.

8. **Empowerment and Control:** Adopting a mindful and intentional approach to eating empowers individuals with diabetes to take control of their health. Understanding the impact of food choices fosters a sense of self-management and confidence in managing diabetes effectively.

The importance of diet in managing diabetes cannot be overstated. A well-thought-out and individualized nutrition plan can contribute significantly to blood sugar control, weight management, heart health, and the prevention of complications. By making informed food choices and embracing a balanced lifestyle, individuals with diabetes can enhance their overall well-being and lead fulfilling, healthy lives.

DIABETES MEAL PLAN

DAY 1:

BREAKFAST: Tomatoes and spinach added to scrambled eggs .Whole grain toast.

Ingredients:

For the Scrambled Eggs:

- 4 large eggs
- 1/4 cup milk (you can use dairy or a dairy-free milk alternative)
- Salt and pepper to taste
- 1 tablespoon olive oil or cooking spray for the pan
- 1 cup fresh spinach leaves, chopped
- 1/2 cup cherry tomatoes, halved
- 2 tablespoons grated Parmesan cheese (optional)

For the Whole Grain Toast:

- 2 slices of whole grain bread
- Butter or margarine (optional)

Instructions:

For the Scrambled Eggs:

1. In a bowl, fully beat together the eggs, milk, salt, and pepper. Set aside.
2. Heat a non-stick skillet over medium heat and add the olive oil or use cooking spray to grease the pan.
3. Add the chopped spinach to the skillet and sauté for 1-2 minutes or until it starts to wilt.
4. Add the halved cherry tomatoes to the pan and continue to cook for another 2-3 minutes until they soften.
5. Pour the egg mixture over the spinach and tomatoes in the pan.
6. Gently stir the mixture with a spatula as it cooks. Cook the eggs for a little while longer, stirring now and then, until they are mostly set but still slightly runny.. This should take about 2-3 minutes.
7. If desired, sprinkle the scrambled eggs with grated Parmesan cheese and continue to cook for another 1-2 minutes, or until the eggs are fully cooked and the cheese is melted.

8. Remove the skillet from the heat when the eggs are cooked to your preferred level of doneness. Be careful not to overcook as the eggs will continue to cook a little from the residual heat.

For the Whole Grain Toast:

1. While the eggs are cooking, toast the whole grain bread slices until they are lightly browned and crisp.
2. Apply a thin coating of margarine or butter.

LUNCH: quinoa, grilled chicken breast, and steamed broccoli.

Ingredients:

For Grilled Chicken:

- 2 boneless, skinless chicken breasts
- 2 tablespoons olive oil
- 1 teaspoon paprika
- 1 teaspoon garlic powder
- 1 teaspoon dried oregano
- Salt and pepper to taste

For Steamed Broccoli:

- 2 cups fresh broccoli florets
- 2 cups water

For Quinoa:

- 1 cup quinoa
- 2 cups water or chicken broth
- Salt to taste

Instructions:

1. Marinate the Chicken: In a bowl, mix olive oil, paprika, garlic powder, dried oregano, salt, and pepper. Coat the chicken breasts with the marinade and let them sit for about 15-30 minutes at room temperature.

2. Preheat the Grill: Adjust the heat on your grill to medium-high (375–400°F/190–200°C). To keep the grates from sticking, make sure they are spotless and lightly oiled.

3. Grill the Chicken: Put the marinated chicken breasts on the grill that has been preheated. Grill for about 6-7 minutes per side or until the internal temperature reaches 165°F (74°C) and the chicken is no longer pink in the center. Depending on the thickness of the chicken breasts, cooking times can change.

4. Steam the Broccoli: While the chicken is grilling, you can steam the broccoli. Heat up a saucepan with two cups of water until it boils. Add the broccoli florets to a steamer basket and place them over the boiling water. Cover with a lid and steam for about 3-4 minutes, or until the broccoli is tender but still vibrant green.

5. Prepare Quinoa: To get rid of any bitter coating, thoroughly rinse the quinoa under cold running water. In a separate saucepan, combine the quinoa and 2 cups of water or chicken broth. When it comes to a boil, add a small pinch of salt. Simmer, covered, over low heat for fifteen minutes, or until all of the liquid has been absorbed. Fluff the quinoa with a fork.

6. Assemble the Dish: Place a portion of cooked quinoa on each plate. Add the grilled chicken breast on top, and arrange the steamed broccoli beside it.

7. Serve and Enjoy: Serve the quinoa, grilled chicken, and steamed broccoli while they are still warm. You can season with additional salt and pepper to taste, or drizzle with a little olive oil or lemon juice if desired.

DINNER: baked salmon served with a little sweet potato and asparagus.

Baked Salmon with Sweet Potato and Asparagus.

Ingredients:

- 4 salmon fillets (about 6-8 ounces each)
- Cut two large sweet potatoes into 1/2-inch cubes after peeling them
- One bundle of raw asparagus, with the woody ends removed
- 2 tablespoons olive oil
- 2 cloves garlic, minced
- 1 teaspoon lemon zest

- 2 tablespoons fresh lemon juice

- 1 teaspoon fresh thyme leaves

- Salt and pepper to taste

- 1/2 teaspoon paprika

- Lemon wedges for garnish

- Fresh parsley for garnish

Instructions:

1. Preheat the oven to 400°F (200°C). A sizable baking sheet should be lightly greased or lined with parchment paper.

2. In a mixing bowl, combine the sweet potato cubes with 1 tablespoon of olive oil, minced garlic, salt, pepper, and paprika. Toss to coat the sweet potatoes evenly. Spread them out on one half of the prepared baking sheet.

3. In another mixing bowl, toss the asparagus with the remaining 1 tablespoon of olive oil, salt, and pepper. The other half of the baking sheet should have them on it.

4. Season the salmon fillets with salt, pepper, lemon zest, and thyme leaves. On top of the asparagus, arrange the salmon fillets.

5. Pour some freshly squeezed lemon juice onto the salmon.

6. Bake in the preheated oven for 15-20 minutes, or until the sweet potatoes are tender and the salmon flakes easily with a fork.

7. If the salmon needs more color, you can switch the oven to the broil setting for the last 2-3 minutes, keeping a close eye to avoid overcooking.

8. Once everything is cooked through and nicely browned, remove from the oven. Add some fresh parsley and lemon wedges as garnish.

9. Serve your baked salmon with sweet potatoes and asparagus hot, and enjoy your delicious and nutritious meal!

DAY 2:

BREAKFAST: Oatmeal with sliced almonds and a sprinkle of cinnamon.

Ingredients:

- 1 cup old-fashioned rolled oats
- 2 cups water
- Pinch of salt
- 1/4 cup sliced almonds
- 1/2 teaspoon ground cinnamon
- 2 tablespoons honey or maple syrup (optional)
- Fresh fruit (e.g., banana slices, berries) for topping (optional)
- Milk (dairy or non-dairy) for serving (optional)

Instructions:

1. **Combine oats and water:** Two cups of water should be brought to a boil in a medium saucepan. Add a pinch of salt to enhance the oatmeal's flavor. Once the water is boiling, stir in 1 cup of old-fashioned rolled oats.

2. **Cook the oats:** After lowering the heat to medium-low, simmer the oats for approximately five minutes, stirring now and then. Adjust the cooking time if you prefer a thicker or thinner oatmeal consistency.

3. **Toast the almonds:** While the oats are cooking, toast the sliced almonds. To accomplish this, put them in a dry skillet and heat it to medium. Stir them frequently until they turn golden and fragrant, which should take about 3-5 minutes. Be careful not to burn them.

4. **Add cinnamon:** When the oats are creamy and have absorbed most of the liquid, stir in 1/2 teaspoon of ground cinnamon. Adjust the amount to taste.

5. **Sweeten (optional):** If you like your oatmeal on the sweeter side, drizzle 2 tablespoons of honey or maple syrup into the oatmeal and mix well. Adjust the sweetness to your preference.

6. **Serve:** Once the oatmeal is cooked to your liking, transfer it to serving bowls.

   Top with the toasted sliced almonds for a delightful crunch and nutty flavor.

7. **Optional toppings:** You can further customize your oatmeal by adding fresh fruit, such as banana slices, berries, or any of your favorite fruits.

   Pour a little milk (dairy or non-dairy) over your oatmeal for added creaminess, if desired.

   Serve your warm oatmeal with sliced almonds and a sprinkle of cinnamon immediately. Enjoy your comforting and nutritious breakfast

LUNCH: Wrap with turkey and avocado on a whole wheat tortilla.

Ingredients:

- 1 whole wheat tortilla
- 4-6 slices of roasted turkey breast
- 1/2 avocado, sliced
- 1/4 cup shredded lettuce
- 2 tablespoons diced tomatoes
- 2 tablespoons thinly sliced red onion

- 2 tablespoons mayonnaise or Greek yogurt

- 1 teaspoon Dijon mustard

- Salt and pepper to taste

Instructions:

1. **Prepare Ingredients:** Position the whole wheat tortilla onto a sanitized surface. In a small bowl, mix together the mayonnaise (or Greek yogurt) and Dijon mustard. Set aside.

2. **Assemble the Wrap:** Spread the mayo and Dijon mixture evenly over the center of the tortilla, leaving a border around the edges. Place the slices of roasted turkey evenly over the sauce.

3. **Add Vegetables:** Layer the sliced avocado, shredded lettuce, diced tomatoes, and thinly sliced red onion on top of the turkey.

4. **Season and Roll:** Over the layered ingredients, add salt and pepper to taste. Starting from one end, tightly roll the tortilla to form a wrap. Make sure the ends are tucked in to prevent fillings from falling out.

5. **Slice and Serve:** Using a sharp knife, slice the wrap diagonally into halves or thirds for easy serving.

6. **Optional: Grill or Toast:** If you prefer a warm wrap, you can lightly grill or toast it on a panini press.

7. **Serve and Enjoy:** Serve your Turkey and Avocado Wrap immediately, either as a wholesome lunch or a satisfying snack.

DINNER: Brown rice with mixed vegetables with stir-fried tofu.

Ingredients:

For the Stir-Fried Tofu:

- Pressed and cubed one block (fourteen ounces) of extra-firm tofu
- 2 tablespoons soy sauce
- 1 tablespoon sesame oil
- 1 tablespoon cornstarch
- 1 tablespoon vegetable oil for frying

For the Brown Rice and Mixed Vegetables:

- 1 cup brown rice (uncooked)

- 2 cups mixed vegetables (broccoli florets, carrots, bell peppers, snap peas, etc.)

- 2 cloves garlic, minced

- 1 tablespoon ginger, grated

- 3 tablespoons soy sauce

- 1 tablespoon sesame oil

- 1 tablespoon vegetable oil

- Salt and pepper to taste

- Green onions, chopped (for garnish, optional)

- Sesame seeds (for garnish, optional)

Instructions:

For the Stir-Fried Tofu:

1. **Press the Tofu:** Press the tofu to remove excess water. You have two options: use a tofu press or cover the tofu block with paper towels and set something heavy on top. Press for at least 15-30 minutes.

2. **Marinate the Tofu:** In a bowl, mix the cubed tofu with soy sauce, sesame oil, and cornstarch. Ensure each piece is coated evenly.

3. **Stir-Fry the Tofu:** Vegetable oil should be heated in a pan over medium-high heat. Add the marinated tofu cubes and stir-fry until they are golden brown and crispy on all sides. Remove and set aside from the pan. For the Brown Rice and Mixed Vegetables:

For Cook Brown Rice:

Follow the package's instructions to prepare the brown rice.

Prepare Vegetables:

In a large pan or wok, heat vegetable oil over medium-high heat.

Add minced garlic and grated ginger, sauté for a minute until fragrant.

1. **Stir-Fry Vegetables:**

When the mixed vegetables are crisp-tender, add them to the pan and stir-fry them.

2. **Combine Tofu, Rice, and Vegetables:** Add the cooked brown rice to the pan with the vegetables. Add the stir-fried tofu to the pan and mix well.

3. **Season the Dish:**
   Cover the mixture with soy sauce and sesame oil. Toss everything together until well combined. Season with salt and pepper to taste.

4. **Garnish and Serve:** If preferred, sprinkle sesame seeds and chopped green onions on top.
   Serve the Brown Rice with Mixed Vegetables and Stir-Fried Tofu hot, and enjoy your nutritious and delicious meal!

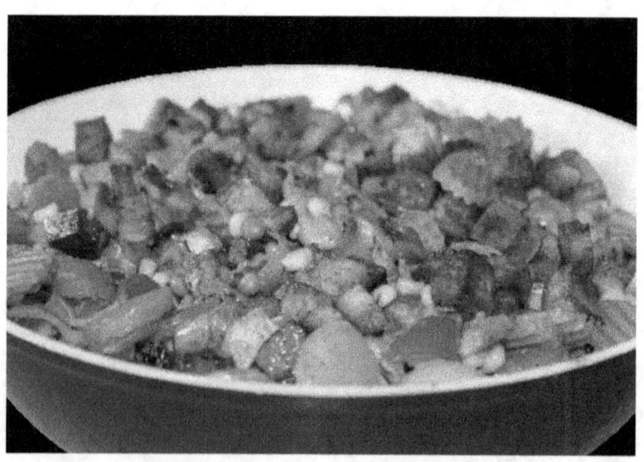

DAY 3:

BREAKFAST:

Plain Greek yogurt with chopped walnuts and a drizzle of honey.

Recipe 1: Classic Greek Yogurt Bowl

Ingredients:

- 1 cup plain Greek yogurt
- 1/4 cup chopped walnuts
- 1-2 tablespoons honey (adjust to taste)

Instructions:

1. Spoon the plain Greek yogurt into a bowl.
2. The walnuts should be evenly distributed throughout the yogurt.
3. Spread honey on top of the walnuts and cream.
4. Use a spoon to gently mix the ingredients, ensuring the honey is evenly distributed.
5. Enjoy this classic and straightforward Greek yogurt bowl!

Recipe 2: Greek Yogurt Parfait

Ingredients:

- 1 cup plain Greek yogurt
- 1/4 cup chopped walnuts
- 1-2 tablespoons honey (adjust to taste)
- 1/2 cup granola
- Fresh berries (optional)

Instructions:

1. In a glass or a bowl, layer half of the plain Greek yogurt.
2. Sprinkle half of the chopped walnuts over the yogurt layer.
3. Drizzle half of the honey over the walnuts.
4. Add a layer of granola on top.
5. Repeat the layers with the remaining yogurt, walnuts, and honey.
6. If desired, top the parfait with fresh berries for added flavor and texture.
7. Serve immediately and enjoy this delightful Greek yogurt parfait!

Lentil soup with a side salad (leafy greens, cherry tomatoes, and balsamic vinaigrette).

For Lentil Soup:

Ingredients:

- One cup of dehydrated green or brown lentils, thoroughly cleaned and drained
- 1 onion, finely chopped
- 2 carrots, diced
- 2 celery stalks, diced
- 3 cloves garlic, minced
- 1 can (14 oz) diced tomatoes
- 6 cups vegetable broth
- 1 teaspoon ground cumin
- 1 teaspoon ground coriander
- 1/2 teaspoon smoked paprika
- Salt and pepper to taste
- 2 tablespoons olive oil
- Fresh cilantro or parsley for garnish (optional)

Instructions:

1. Lightly warm the olive oil in a large pot over medium heat. Add the chopped onion, carrots, and celery. The vegetables should be sautéed for about five minutes, or until they are tender.

2. Add the cumin, ground coriander, smoked paprika, and finely chopped garlic. Stir well to coat the vegetables in the spices and cook for an additional 2 minutes.

3. After adding the rinsed lentils, pour in the vegetable broth. After bringing the soup to a boil, lower the heat to a simmer, cover it, and let it cook for 25 to 30 minutes, or until the lentils are soft.

4. Add the diced tomatoes and taste and adjust the seasoning with salt and pepper. Simmer for an additional 10 minutes.

5. Before serving, garnish with fresh parsley or cilantro, if preferred.

For Leafy greens, cherry tomatoes, and balsamic vinaigrette on a side salad:

Ingredients:

- 4 cups mixed leafy greens (e.g., spinach, arugula, or mixed salad greens)
- 1 cup cherry tomatoes, halved
- 1/4 cup balsamic vinaigrette dressing
- Salt and pepper to taste

Instructions:

1. In a large bowl, combine the mixed leafy greens and cherry tomatoes.
2. Drizzle the balsamic vinaigrette over the salad and toss until well coated.
3. Add pepper and salt according to taste.

DINNER:

Quinoa and sautéed spinach paired with grilled shrimp.

Grilled Shrimp:

Ingredients:

- 1 pound large shrimp, peeled and deveined
- 2 tablespoons olive oil
- 2 cloves garlic, minced
- 1 teaspoon smoked paprika
- Salt and pepper to taste
- Fresh lemon wedges for serving

Instructions:

1. In a bowl, combine the shrimp with olive oil, minced garlic, smoked paprika, salt, and pepper. Until the shrimp are coated evenly, toss them.
2. Turn the heat up to medium-high on a grill or grill pan.

3. Thread the shrimp onto skewers or place them directly on the grill.

4. Grill the shrimp for 2-3 minutes per side or until they are opaque and cooked through.

5. Remove from the grill and squeeze fresh lemon juice over the grilled shrimp.

Quinoa and Sautéed Spinach:

Ingredients:

- 1 cup quinoa, rinsed
- 2 cups water or vegetable broth
- 2 tablespoons olive oil
- 1 onion, finely chopped
- 3 cups fresh spinach, washed and chopped
- Salt and pepper to taste
- Lemon zest for garnish

Instructions:

1. Once the quinoa is cooked and the water has been absorbed, reduce the heat to low, cover, and simmer for 15 to 20 minutes.

2. Olive oil should be heated to medium heat in a big skillet. When the onion is soft, add it chopped and sauté it

3. Toss in the chopped spinach and cook until it wilts in the skillet.

4. Stir in the cooked quinoa and toss until well combined. Add salt and water to taste when preparing.

5. Garnish with lemon zest before serving.

1. VEGGIE OMELETTE WITH AVOCADO

Introduction:

Start your day with a protein-packed omelette filled with colorful veggies and topped with creamy avocado for a satisfying and diabetes-friendly breakfast.

Ingredients:

- 2 eggs
- 1/4 cup diced bell peppers
- 1/4 cup diced tomatoes
- 1/4 cup diced onions
- Salt and pepper to taste
- 1/2 avocado, sliced

Preparation:

1. In a bowl, whisk together eggs and add pepper and salt to taste.

2. Heat a non-stick skillet over medium heat, add the veggies, and cook until softened.

3. Pour the whisked eggs over the veggies, cook until set, and fold the omelette.
4. Top with sliced avocado and serve.

Prep Time: 15 minutes

2. BERRIES AND ALMONDS PAIRED WITH A GREEK YOGURT PARFAIT

Introduction:

A refreshing and protein-rich parfait with Greek yogurt, fresh berries, and crunchy almonds—perfect for a quick and healthy diabetic breakfast.

Ingredients:

- 1 cup Greek yogurt (unsweetened)
- 1/2 cup mixed berries (blueberries, strawberries)
- 2 tablespoons chopped almonds
- 1 teaspoon honey (optional)

Preparation:

1. Arrange almonds, berries, and Greek yogurt in a bowl or glass.
2. Drizzle with honey if desired.

3.   Repeat the layers.
4.   Serve chilled.

Prep Time: 10 minutes

3. SPINACH AND FETA EGG MUFFINS

Introduction:

These portable egg muffins are loaded with spinach and feta, providing a convenient and low-carb option for a diabetic-friendly breakfast.

Ingredients:

- 4 eggs
- 1 cup chopped spinach
- 1/4 cup crumbled feta cheese
- Salt and pepper to taste

Preparation:

1.   Preheat the oven to 350°F (175°C).
2.   Add salt and pepper to a bowl and whisk the eggs.
3.   Mix in chopped spinach and feta.
4.   Pour the mixture into muffin cups and bake for 15-20 minutes until set.

Prep Time: 25 minutes

4. CHIA SEED PUDDING WITH ALMOND MILK

Introduction:

A nutrient-packed chia seed pudding made with almond milk, topped with fresh berries—high in fiber and suitable for a diabetic breakfast.

Ingredients:

- 2 tablespoons chia seeds
- 1/2 cup unsweetened almond milk
- 1/2 teaspoon vanilla extract
- Fresh berries for topping

Preparation:

1. Mix chia seeds, almond milk, and vanilla extract in a bowl.
2. Chill for a minimum of two hours or leave it in overnight.
3. Top with fresh berries before serving.

Prep Time: 2 hours (including chilling time)

Ingredients:

- 1 cup diced fresh pineapple
- 1 cup coconut milk (can use light or full-fat)
- 1/4 cup chia seeds
- One tablespoon of maple syrup or honey (optional; taste and adjust)
- 1/4 teaspoon vanilla extract
- Shredded coconut and additional pineapple chunks for topping (optional)

Instructions:

1. In a blender or food processor, blend 3/4 cup of the diced pineapple until smooth.

2. In a mixing bowl, combine the blended pineapple, coconut milk, chia seeds, honey or maple syrup (if using), and vanilla extract. Mix well until thoroughly combined.

3. To keep the chia seeds from clumping, let the mixture sit for about five minutes before stirring it again. Let it sit for another 5-10 minutes and stir once more.

4. Cover the bowl and refrigerate the mixture for at least 2 hours or overnight to allow the chia seeds to expand and create a pudding-like consistency. Stir occasionally during this time.

5. When ready to serve, give the pudding a final stir. Divide it into serving bowls or jars.

6. Top each portion with the remaining diced pineapple, shredded coconut, and any additional pineapple chunks for garnish.

7. Enjoy your pineapple coconut chia pudding as a refreshing and nutritious breakfast!

Prep Time: 45 minutes

6. ALMOND FLOUR PANCAKES

Introduction:

Fluffy and nutty almond flour pancakes, a low-carb alternative to traditional pancakes, served with sugar-free syrup.

Ingredients:

- 1 cup almond flour
- 2 eggs
- 1/4 cup unsweetened almond milk

- 1 teaspoon baking powder
- Sugar-free syrup for serving

Preparation:

1. In a bowl, whisk together almond flour, eggs, almond milk, and baking powder.
2. Heat a skillet, pour batter to make pancakes, and cook until bubbles form.
3. Flip and cook until golden brown.
4. Serve with sugar-free syrup.

Prep Time: 20 minutes

7. SMOKED SALMON AND AVOCADO WRAP

Introduction:

A protein-rich wrap with smoked salmon and creamy avocado, providing healthy fats and omega-3s for a diabetic-friendly breakfast.

Ingredients:

- 1 whole-grain or low-carb wrap
- 2 ounces smoked salmon
- 1/2 avocado, sliced
- Fresh dill for garnish

Preparation:

1. Lay the wrap flat.
2. Arrange smoked salmon and sliced avocado.
3. Garnish with fresh dill.
4. Roll the wrap and slice.

Prep Time: 10 minutes

8. **SWEET POTATO HASH WITH TURKEY SAUSAGE**

Introduction:

A hearty and flavorful sweet potato hash with lean turkey sausage, offering a balanced breakfast for those managing diabetes.

Ingredients:

- 1 medium sweet potato, diced
- 4 ounces lean turkey sausage, crumbled
- 1/2 onion, diced
- 1 bell pepper, diced
- 1 tablespoon olive oil
- Salt and pepper to taste

Preparation:

1. Warm up the olive oil in a skillet using a medium flame.
2. Add diced sweet potato, onion, and bell pepper. Cook until sweet potatoes are tender.
3. Add crumbled turkey sausage and cook until browned.
4. Season with salt and pepper.

Prep Time: 30 minutes

9. MUSHROOM AND SPINACH SCRAMBLE

Introduction:

A quick and nutritious egg scramble with sautéed mushrooms and spinach, providing vitamins and minerals for a diabetic-friendly breakfast.

Ingredients:

- 3 eggs
- 1 cup sliced mushrooms
- 1 cup fresh spinach
- 1 tablespoon olive oil
- Salt and pepper to taste

Preparation:

1. In a skillet, sauté mushrooms in olive oil until browned.
2. Cook until the fresh spinach wilts after adding it.
3. Whisk eggs and pour into the skillet.
4. Scramble until eggs are cooked.
5. Season with salt and pepper.

Prep Time: 15 minutes

10. BERRY AND ALMOND SMOOTHIE BOWL

Introduction:

A vibrant and nutrient-packed smoothie bowl with mixed berries, almond milk, and topped with crunchy almonds—a delicious and diabetes-friendly breakfast option.

Ingredients:

- One cup of mixed berries, including raspberries, blueberries, and strawberries
- 1/2 cup unsweetened almond milk
- 1 tablespoon almond butter
- 2 tablespoons sliced almonds
- Chia seeds for garnish

Preparation:

1. Blend mixed berries, almond milk, and almond butter until smooth.
2. Transfer into a bowl, then sprinkle chia seeds and sliced almonds on top.

Prep Time: 10 minutes

1. GRILLED CHICKEN AND VEGETABLE SALAD

Introduction:

This refreshing salad is a perfect low-carb option for diabetics. Packed with lean protein and colorful veggies, it's both nutritious and delicious.

Ingredients:

- 1 boneless, skinless chicken breast
- 2 cups mixed salad greens
- 1 cup cherry tomatoes, halved
- 1 cucumber, sliced
- 1/4 cup red onion, thinly sliced
- 2 tablespoons olive oil
- 1 tablespoon balsamic vinegar
- Salt and pepper to taste

Preparation:

1. Use salt and pepper to season the chicken breast.

2. Grill the chicken until fully cooked, approximately 6-8 minutes per side.

3. Thinly slice the chicken that has been grilled.

4. In a large bowl, combine salad greens, cherry tomatoes, cucumber, and red onion.

5. Add balsamic vinegar and olive oil to the salad and toss.

6. Top the salad with grilled chicken strips.

7. Serve immediately.

Prep Time: 20 minutes

2. QUINOA AND ROASTED VEGETABLE BOWL

Introduction:

Quinoa is a fantastic option for a diabetic-friendly lunch because it's high in protein and fiber. This bowl is filled with colorful roasted vegetables for added vitamins and minerals.

Ingredients:

- 1 cup quinoa, rinsed
- Two cups of mixed veggies, including cherry tomatoes, zucchini, and bell peppers
- 2 tablespoons olive oil
- 1 teaspoon dried oregano
- 1 teaspoon garlic powder
- Salt and pepper to taste
- Fresh parsley for garnish

Preparation:

1. Cook quinoa according to package instructions.
2. Preheat the oven to 400°F (200°C).
3. Toss the mixed vegetables with olive oil, oregano, garlic powder, salt, and pepper.
4. After spreading out on a baking sheet, roast the vegetables for 20 to 25 minutes, or until they are soft.
5. Fluff the cooked quinoa with a fork and divide it among serving bowls.
6. Top with roasted vegetables and garnish with fresh parsley.

Prep Time: 30 minutes

3. SALMON AND ASPARAGUS FOIL PACKETS

Introduction:

This simple-to-prepare dinner in a foil packet is high in omega-3 fatty acids and suitable for diabetics. The salmon is kept moist and the flavors are sealed in the foil packets.

Ingredients:

- 2 salmon fillets
- 1 bunch asparagus, trimmed
- 2 tablespoons olive oil
- 1 lemon, sliced
- 2 cloves garlic, minced
- Salt and pepper to taste
- Fresh dill for garnish

Preparation:

1. Preheat the oven to 400°F (200°C).
2. Line a piece of foil with each salmon fillet.
3. Arrange asparagus around the salmon.

4. Season the salmon and asparagus with a drizzle of olive oil.

5. Sprinkle minced garlic, salt, and pepper.

6. Place lemon slices on top.

7. Fold the foil to create packets, ensuring they are sealed.

8. Bake for 15-20 minutes.

9. Garnish with fresh dill before serving.

Prep Time: 25 minutes

4. LENTIL AND VEGETABLE STEW

Introduction:

This hearty stew is high in fiber and plant-based protein, making it an excellent choice for diabetics. Packed with vegetables, it's a nutritious and satisfying lunch option.

Ingredients:

- One cup of rinsed and dry brown or green lentils
- 4 cups vegetable broth
- 1 onion, diced
- 2 carrots, diced
- 2 celery stalks, chopped
- 2 cloves garlic, minced
- 1 can (14 oz) diced tomatoes
- 1 teaspoon ground cumin
- 1 teaspoon smoked paprika
- Salt and pepper to taste
- Fresh parsley for garnish

Preparation:

1. Sauté the celery, carrots, and onions in a big pot until they are tender.
2. Add garlic, cumin, and smoked paprika, stirring for 1-2 minutes.
3. After adding the lentils, pour in the vegetable broth.
4. Bring to a boil and simmer over low heat for 25 to 30 minutes, or until the lentils are tender.
5. Add diced tomatoes, salt, and pepper. Simmer for an additional 10 minutes.
6. Garnish with fresh parsley before serving.

Prep Time: 45 minutes

5. TURKEY AND AVOCADO WRAP

Introduction:

A low-carb and protein-packed lunch, this turkey and avocado wrap is a quick and easy option for those busy days.

Ingredients:

- 4 large lettuce leaves (butter or iceberg)
- 8 slices turkey breast
- 1 avocado, sliced
- 1 tomato, sliced
- 1/4 cup Greek yogurt
- 1 tablespoon Dijon mustard
- Salt and pepper to taste

Preparation:

1. In a small bowl, mix Greek yogurt, Dijon mustard, salt, and pepper.
2. Lay out the lettuce leaves and spread the yogurt mixture on each leaf.
3. Place two slices of turkey on each leaf.
4. Add avocado and tomato slices.

5. Roll the lettuce leaves to form wraps.

6. Secure with toothpicks if needed.

7. Serve immediately.

Prep Time: 15 minutes

6. EGG SALAD LETTUCE WRAPS

Introduction:

An excellent source of protein, these egg salad lettuce wraps are light, flavorful, and perfect for a diabetic-friendly lunch.

Ingredients:

- 4 large lettuce leaves
- 6 hard-boiled eggs, chopped
- 1/4 cup mayonnaise (or Greek yogurt for a lighter option)
- 1 tablespoon Dijon mustard
- 2 green onions, finely chopped
- Salt and pepper to taste
- Paprika for garnish

Preparation:

1. In a bowl, combine chopped eggs, mayonnaise, Dijon mustard, and green onions.
2. Mix until well combined. Add salt and pepper to taste.
3. Spoon the egg salad onto each lettuce leaf.
4. Sprinkle paprika for garnish.
5. Serve immediately.

Prep Time: 20 minutes

7. SHRIMP AND BROCCOLI STIR-FRY

Introduction:

This quick and flavorful shrimp and broccoli stir-fry is low in carbs and high in protein, making it an excellent choice for a diabetic lunch.

Ingredients:

- 1 pound shrimp, peeled and deveined
- 2 cups broccoli florets
- 1 bell pepper, sliced
- 2 tablespoons soy sauce

- 1 tablespoon sesame oil
- 2 cloves garlic, minced
- 1 teaspoon ginger, grated
- 1 tablespoon olive oil
- Sesame seeds for garnish

Preparation:

1. Olive oil should be heated to medium-high temperature in a wok or big skillet.
2. Add shrimp and stir-fry until pink and opaque. Extract and set aside from the pan.
3. In the same pan, add broccoli and bell pepper. Stir-fry for 3-4 minutes.
4. Add garlic and ginger, stir-frying for an additional 1-2 minutes.
5. Return the cooked shrimp to the pan.
6. Drizzle the mixture with sesame oil and soy sauce.. Toss until everything is well coated.
7. Garnish with sesame seeds before serving.

Prep Time: 20 minutes

8. CAULIFLOWER FRIED RICE WITH CHICKEN

Introduction:

A low-carb alternative to traditional fried rice, this cauliflower fried rice with chicken is a tasty and satisfying diabetic-friendly lunch.

Ingredients:

- 1 head cauliflower, grated
- 1 cup cooked chicken breast, diced
- One cup of mixed veggies (corn, carrots, and peas)
- 2 eggs, beaten
- 3 tablespoons soy sauce
- 1 tablespoon sesame oil
- 2 green onions, chopped
- 1 tablespoon olive oil

Preparation:

1. Fill a large skillet with olive oil and heat over medium heat.
2. Add grated cauliflower and cook for 5-7 minutes, stirring occasionally.
3. Push cauliflower to the side of the pan and pour beaten eggs into the empty side.
4. Scramble the eggs and mix with the cauliflower.
5. Add cooked chicken, mixed vegetables, soy sauce, and sesame oil. Stir well.
6. Cook until everything is thoroughly heated, about 5 more minutes.
7. Before serving, sprinkle some chopped green onions on top

Prep Time: 25 minutes

9. SPINACH AND FETA STUFFED CHICKEN BREAST

Introduction:

This stuffed chicken breast is not only diabetic-friendly but also elegant enough for a special lunch. The combination of spinach and feta adds flavor without compromising on nutrition.

Ingredients:

- 2 boneless, skinless chicken breasts
- 2 cups fresh spinach, chopped
- 1/2 cup feta cheese, crumbled
- 2 cloves garlic, minced
- 1 tablespoon olive oil
- Salt and pepper to taste
- Toothpicks for securing

Preparation:

1. Preheat the oven to 375°F (190°C).
2. Heat the olive oil in a skillet over a medium heat source.

3. Add minced garlic and sauté until fragrant.

4. Add chopped spinach and cook until wilted.

5. Remove the skillet from heat and stir in feta cheese.

6. Cut a pocket into each chicken breast.

7. Stuff the chicken breasts with the spinach and feta mixture.

8. Secure with toothpicks.

9. Apply salt and pepper to the chicken's exterior.

10. Once the chicken is thoroughly cooked, bake it for 25 to 30 minutes.

Prep Time: 35 minutes

10. BLACK BEAN AND VEGETABLE QUESADILLAS

Introduction:

These black bean and vegetable quesadillas are a delicious and satisfying lunch option for diabetics, offering a balance of protein, fiber, and flavor.

Ingredients:

- 4 whole wheat tortillas
- One can (15 oz) of rinsed and drained black beans

- 1 cup bell peppers, thinly sliced
- 1 cup zucchini, grated
- One cup of shredded cheese, either Mexican blend or cheddar
- 1 teaspoon cumin
- 1 teaspoon chili powder
- Olive oil for cooking

Preparation:

1. In a bowl, mix black beans, bell peppers, zucchini, cumin, and chili powder.
2. Lay out the tortillas and spread the bean and vegetable mixture on half of each tortilla.
3. Sprinkle shredded cheese over the mixture.
4. Fold the tortillas in half, creating quesadillas.
5. In a skillet over medium heat, the olive oil should be warmed.
6. Once the cheese has melted and the tortillas have turned golden brown, cook the quesadillas for two to three minutes on each side.
7. Cut into wedges and serve with salsa or Greek yogurt.

Prep Time: 20 minutes

1. GRILLED CHICKEN WITH HERBS AND SPICES AND ROASTED VEGGIES.

Introduction:

This diabetic-friendly dinner is light, flavorful, and low in carbohydrates. The grilled lemon herb chicken pairs perfectly with a medley of roasted vegetables.

Ingredients:

- 4 boneless, skinless chicken breasts
- 1 lemon, juiced and zested
- 2 tablespoons olive oil
- 2 teaspoons dried herbs (rosemary, thyme, oregano)
- Salt and pepper to taste
- Four cups of mixed veggies, including cherry tomatoes, bell peppers, and zucchini

Preparation:

1. In a bowl, combine lemon juice, lemon zest, olive oil, dried herbs, salt, and pepper.
2. For a minimum of half an hour, marinate chicken breasts in the mixture.
3. Preheat the grill.
4. Cook the chicken for 6 to 8 minutes on each side, or until it's done.
5. Combine salt, pepper, and olive oil with the mixed vegetables.
6. Roast the vegetables in the oven at 400°F (200°C) for 20-25 minutes.
7. Serve grilled chicken on a bed of roasted vegetables.

Prep Time: 45 minutes

2. SALMON AND QUINOA STUFFED BELL PEPPERS

Introduction:

These stuffed bell peppers are not only visually appealing but also a nutritious, low-carb dinner option for individuals managing diabetes.

Ingredients:

- 4 bell peppers, halved and seeds removed
- 1 cup quinoa, cooked
- Two 14-oz cans of drained and flaked salmon
- 1 cup cherry tomatoes, halved
- 1/4 cup feta cheese, crumbled
- 1 teaspoon dried dill
- Salt and pepper to taste
- Olive oil for drizzling

Preparation:

1. Preheat the oven to 375°F (190°C).
2. Place bell peppers on a baking sheet.
3. In a bowl, combine quinoa, salmon, cherry tomatoes, feta cheese, dried dill, salt, and pepper.

4. Place the quinoa and salmon mixture inside each half of a bell pepper.

5. Drizzle with olive oil.

6. Once the peppers are soft, bake for 25 to 30 minutes.

7. Serve warm.

Prep Time: 40 minutes

3. VEGETARIAN CHICKPEA AND SPINACH CURRY

Introduction:

This hearty and flavorful chickpea and spinach curry is rich in plant-based protein and fiber, making it a satisfying option for a diabetic dinner.

Ingredients:

- Two cans (15 oz each) of rinsed and drained chickpeas

- 1 onion, finely chopped

- 2 tomatoes, diced

- 3 cups fresh spinach

- 1 can (14 oz) coconut milk

- 2 tablespoons curry powder
- 1 teaspoon turmeric

  1 teaspoon cumin
- Salt and pepper to taste
- Olive oil for cooking

Preparation:

1. Chop the onion and sauté it in olive oil in a big pan until it becomes transparent.
2. Add curry powder, turmeric, and cumin. Stir for 1-2 minutes.
3. Cook the chopped tomatoes until they begin to soften.
4. Bring the mixture to a simmer after adding the coconut milk.
5. Add chickpeas and simmer for 15-20 minutes.
6. Stir in fresh spinach until wilted.
7. Season with salt and pepper.
8. Serve over brown rice or cauliflower rice.

Prep Time: 30 minutes

4. TURKEY AND VEGETABLE STIR-FRY WITH CAULIFLOWER RICE

Introduction:

This dish, which is served over cauliflower rice and includes lean turkey and a rainbow of vegetables, is a low-carb substitute for traditional stir-fry and is suitable for diabetics.

Ingredients:

- 1 pound ground turkey
- 1 cauliflower, grated (for cauliflower rice)
- Two cups of mixed veggies, such as bell peppers, broccoli, and snap peas
- 3 tablespoons low-sodium soy sauce
- 1 tablespoon sesame oil
- 2 cloves garlic, minced
- 1 teaspoon ginger, grated
- Green onions for garnish

Preparation:

1. Cook the ground turkey until it's cooked through in a big skillet.
2. Add minced garlic and grated ginger, stirring for 1-2 minutes.
3. Add mixed vegetables and stir-fry until crisp-tender.
4. In a separate pan, sauté cauliflower rice until tender.
5. Mix soy sauce and sesame oil, then pour over the turkey and vegetable mixture.
6. Stir well to combine.
7. Serve the stir-fry over cauliflower rice.
8. Garnish with chopped green onions.

Prep Time: 30 minutes

5. MEDITERRANEAN BAKED COD WITH TOMATO AND OLIVE RELISH

Introduction:

This Mediterranean-inspired baked cod is light, heart-healthy, and bursting with flavors. Relish of tomatoes and olives gives it a cool feel.

Ingredients:

- 4 cod fillets
- 2 cups cherry tomatoes, halved
- 1/2 cup Kalamata olives, sliced
- 2 tablespoons capers
- 2 cloves garlic, minced
- 1 lemon, sliced
- 2 tablespoons olive oil
- 1 teaspoon dried oregano
- Salt and pepper to taste

Preparation:

1. Preheat the oven to 375°F (190°C).
2. Place cod fillets in a baking dish.

3. In a bowl, combine cherry tomatoes, Kalamata olives, capers, minced garlic, lemon slices, olive oil, oregano, salt, and pepper.

4. Spoon the tomato and olive relish over the cod fillets.

5. Fish should flake easily with a fork after 20 to 25 minutes in the oven.

6. Serve with a side of steamed vegetables.

Prep Time: 30 minutes

6. VEGETABLE AND LENTIL SOUP

Introduction:

A comforting and nutritious option, this vegetable and lentil soup is high in fiber and protein, making it an ideal dinner for those managing diabetes.

Ingredients:

- One cup of rinsed, dried lentils (brown or green)
- 1 onion, diced
- 2 carrots, diced
- 2 celery stalks, chopped
- 3 cloves garlic, minced

- 1 can (14 oz) diced tomatoes
- 6 cups vegetable broth
- 1 teaspoon dried thyme
- 1 teaspoon paprika
- Salt and pepper to taste
- Fresh parsley for garnish

Preparation:

1. Add the onions, carrots, and celery to a large pot and sauté until softened.
2. Add minced garlic, thyme, and paprika, stirring for 1-2 minutes.
3. Pour in vegetable broth and add lentils.
4. The lentils should be soft after 25 to 30 minutes of simmering on low heat after bringing to a boil.
5. Add diced tomatoes, salt, and pepper. Simmer for an additional 10 minutes.
6. Garnish with fresh parsley before serving.
7. Serve with a slice of whole-grain bread.

Prep Time: 45 minutes

7. CHICKEN AND BROCCOLI QUICHE WITH ALMOND FLOUR CRUST

Introduction:

This almond flour crust quiche is a low-carb, high-protein dinner option. The combination of chicken and broccoli makes it both delicious and nutritious.

Ingredients:

For the Crust:

- 1.5 cups almond flour
- 1/4 cup melted butter
- 1 egg
- 1/2 teaspoon salt

For the Filling:

- 2 cups cooked chicken breast, shredded
- 1.5 cups broccoli florets, blanched
- 1 cup shredded cheddar cheese
- 4 large eggs
- 1 cup unsweetened almond milk
- Salt and pepper to taste

Preparation:

For the Crust:

1. Preheat the oven to 350°F (175°C).
2. In a bowl, combine almond flour, melted butter, egg, and salt.
3. Construct the crust by pressing the mixture into a pie dish.
4. Bake for 10 minutes.

For the Filling:

1. In a bowl, whisk together eggs and almond milk.
2. Arrange the pre-baked crust in layers, top with cheddar cheese, blanched broccoli, and shredded chicken.
3. Pour the egg and almond milk mixture over the filling.
4. Once the quiche has set, bake it for 30 to 35 minutes.
5. After ten minutes of cooling, cut into slices.

Prep Time: 45 minutes

8. SHRIMP AND AVOCADO SALAD WITH LIME VINAIGRETTE

Introduction:

This refreshing shrimp and avocado salad is a light and satisfying dinner option. The lime vinaigrette adds a zesty kick to enhance the flavors.

Ingredients:

- 1 pound shrimp, peeled and deveined
- 2 avocados, diced
- 1 cup cherry tomatoes, halved
- 1 cucumber, sliced
- 1/4 cup red onion, thinly sliced
- 1/4 cup fresh cilantro, chopped
- 2 tablespoons olive oil
- 2 limes, juiced
- Salt and pepper to taste

Preparation:

1. In a pot, bring water to a boil and cook shrimp until pink and opaque.
2. In a large bowl, combine shrimp, diced avocados, cherry tomatoes, cucumber, red onion, and cilantro.
3. Mix the olive oil, lime juice, salt, and pepper in a small bowl.
4. Drizzle the lime vinaigrette over the salad and toss gently to combine.
5. Before serving, let the food cool for at least half an hour in the refrigerator.
6. Serve over a bed of mixed greens or with a side of quinoa.

Prep Time: 30 minutes

9. EGGPLANT AND CHICKPEA CURRY

Introduction:

This hearty eggplant and chickpea curry is a flavorful and filling option for a diabetic-friendly dinner. The combination of spices creates a satisfying dish.

Ingredients:

- 1 large eggplant, diced
- One can (15 oz) of rinsed and drained chickpeas
- 1 onion, finely chopped
- 2 tomatoes, diced
- 3 cloves garlic, minced
- 1 teaspoon ground cumin
- 1 teaspoon ground coriander
- 1 teaspoon turmeric
- 1 teaspoon paprika
- 1 can (14 oz) coconut milk
- Salt and pepper to taste
- Fresh cilantro for garnish

Preparation:

1. Chop the onion and sauté it in olive oil in a big pan until it becomes transparent.
2. Add minced garlic, ground cumin, ground coriander, turmeric, and paprika. Stir for 1-2 minutes.
3. Add diced eggplant and cook until softened.

4. After adding the coconut milk, boil the mixture.

5. Add chickpeas and diced tomatoes. Simmer for 15-20 minutes.

6. Season with salt and pepper.

7. Garnish with fresh cilantro before serving.

8. Serve with brown rice or cauliflower rice.

Prep Time: 40 minutes

10. ZUCCHINI NOODLES WITH PESTO AND GRILLED CHICKEN

Introduction:

A low-carb alternative to pasta, these zucchini noodles are paired with homemade pesto and grilled chicken for a light and flavorful diabetic-friendly dinner.

Ingredients:

- 4 zucchinis, spiralized into noodles

- 2 boneless, skinless chicken breasts

- 1 cup fresh basil leaves

- 1/2 cup grated Parmesan cheese

- 1/4 cup pine nuts

- 2 cloves garlic
- 1/2 cup olive oil
- Salt and pepper to taste
- Cherry tomatoes for garnish

Preparation:

1. Preheat the grill.
2. Season chicken breasts with salt and pepper and grill until fully cooked.
3. In a food processor, combine basil, Parmesan cheese, pine nuts, and garlic. Pulse until finely chopped.
4. With the processor running, slowly add olive oil until the pesto reaches a smooth consistency.
5. In a pan, sauté zucchini noodles until just tender.
6. Slice grilled chicken into strips.
7. Toss zucchini noodles with pesto and top with grilled chicken.
8. Garnish with cherry tomatoes.
9. Serve immediately.

Prep Time: 30 minutes

CONCLUSION

In closing, this diabetes recipes diet cookbook is more than a compilation of culinary creations—it's a beacon of hope and empowerment for those navigating life with diabetes. Through the artful curation of flavorful, diabetes-friendly recipes, it unveils a path to embrace food as a powerful ally in managing this condition.

Within these pages lie not just meals, but a celebration of health, innovation, and the joy of savoring delicious dishes while keeping blood sugar in check. This cookbook is a testament to the fusion of culinary expertise and nutritional wisdom, transforming the dietary landscape for those seeking balance and control.

As you embark on this gastronomic journey, remember that every recipe represents not only a delightful culinary experience but also a step toward a healthier, more vibrant life. May these recipes not just nourish your body but also invigorate your spirit, inspiring a fulfilling and flavorful journey towards wellness. Here's to embracing a delicious life while managing diabetes with grace and confidence.

9 798878 528986